DIVERTICULITIS

THINGS YOU SHOULD KNOW
(QUESTIONS AND ANSWERS)

By Rumi Michael Leigh

Introduction

I would like to thank and congratulate you for purchasing this book, " *Diverticulitis, things you should know (questions and answers)*" series.

This book will help you understand, revise and have a good general knowledge and keywords of Diverticulitis and how it affects the lives of people who suffer from this disease.

Thanks again for purchasing this book, I hope you enjoy it!

Chapter 1

1) What is diverticulitis ?

- Diverticulitis is an inflammation of the diverticula.

2) What is diverticulum ?

- Diverticulum is a single pocket on the digestive tract.

3) What are diverticula ?

- Diverticula are pockets around the digestive tract.

4) What is the medical term for diverticulum ?

- The medical term for diverticulum is hernia.

5) What are the risk factors for diverticulum ?

- The risk factors for diverticulum are diet (low fiber), age, sedentary lifestyle, insufficient hydration, stress, and heredity.

6) What is a true diverticulum ?

- In a true diverticulum, all the layers of the walls of the colon are involved.

7) What is a false diverticulum ?

- In a false diverticulum, only the mucosa and the submucosa of the walls of the colon are involved.

8) What is a sedentary lifestyle ?

- A sedentary lifestyle is a lifestyle with no or very little physical activity by an individual.

9) Do diverticula cause symptoms ?

- No, diverticula do not cause symptoms.

Chapter 2

1) What is another name for the large intestine ?

- The colon is another name for the large intestine.

2) Give another name for the serosa of the digestive tract.

- Another name for the serosa of the digestive tract is the peritoneum.

3) What are the layers of the digestive tract ?

- The layers of the digestive tract are the mucosa, the submucosa, the muscularis and the serosa.

4) What could be the result of a low fiber diet ?

- A low fiber diet could lead to constipation.

5) What is an abscess ?

- An abscess is a collection of pus in the tissue of the body.

6) What is the danger of an abscess in the colon ?

- An abscess in the colon can lead to a rupture that can cause peritonitis.

7) What is peritonitis ?

- Peritonitis is the inflammation of the peritoneum.

8) Is peritonitis life-threatening ?

-   Yes, peritonitis is a life-threatening condition.

9) What kind of hemorrhage is caused by peritonitis?

-   The type of hemorrhage caused by peritonitis is gastrointestinal bleeding.

10) What is hematochezia ?

-   Hematochezia is the presence of fresh brightly red blood in stool.

Chapter 3

1) What are the parts of the colon ?

- The parts of the colon include the caecum, the ascending colon, the transverse colon, the descending colon, the rectum, and the sigmoid.

2) What part of the colon has the smallest diameter?

- The sigmoid has the smallest diameter.

3) What part of the colon is subject to the highest pressure ?

- The sigmoid is subject to the highest pressure since it has the smallest diameter in the colon.

4) What is a colovesical fistula ?

- A colovesical fistula is a connection between the colon and the bladder due to a rupture of a diverticula.

5) What is colonoscopy ?

- Colonoscopy is a medical examination of the colon.

6) What is the advantage of colonoscopy ?

- A colonoscopy allows the doctor to see clearly all the parts of the colon in real time.

7) What is a common risk of performing colonoscopy on a patient ?

- A common risk of performing colonoscopy on a patient is the risk of perforation.

8) What is a CT scan ?

- A CT scan is an X-ray and a computer exam that allows the doctor to see the inside of a patient's body.

9) In what situation can a CT scan be recommended by a physician instead of a colonoscopy ?

- If the bowels are too inflamed and there is a high risk of infection, the physician may recommend a CT scan instead of a colonoscopy.

10) What is Barium enema ?

- Barium enema is an X-ray exam of the colon.

Chapter 4

1) What is diverticulosis ?

- Diverticulosis is a set of diverticula.

2) What is the main cause of diverticulosis ?

- The main cause of diverticulosis is unknown.

3) Can diverticulosis be found everywhere in the intestine ?

- Yes, diverticulosis can be found everywhere in the intestine.

4) Where is diverticulosis most commonly found in the intestine ?

- Diverticulosis is most commonly found in the sigmoid colon.

5) Is diverticulosis symptomatic or asymptomatic ?

- Diverticulosis is usually asymptomatic.

6) How is diverticulosis diagnosed ?

- Diverticulosis can be diagnosed by colonoscopy, a CT-scan, and barium enema.

7) What are the complications of diverticulosis ?

- The complications of diverticulosis are bleeding, diverticulitis, fistula, a decrease in diameter of the bowel walls, etc.

8) Does diverticulosis always lead to diverticulitis ?

- No, not all diverticulosis cases lead to diverticulitis.

Chapter 5

1) What are the complications of diverticulitis ?

- The complications of diverticulitis are pain, peritonitis, fever, constipation, etc.

2) What are the treatments of diverticulitis ?

- The treatment of diverticulitis are antibiotics, abscess drainage, surgery, and colostomy.

3) What part of the body does pain usually occur during diverticulitis ?

- Pain usually occurs on the left iliac fossa during diverticulitis.

4) Why does pain often occur on the left iliac fossa during diverticulitis ?

- Pain often occurs on the left fossa during diverticulitis because that is the position of the sigmoid.

5) What are the signs and symptoms of diverticulitis?

- The signs and symptoms of diverticulitis are inflammation, infection, nausea, vomiting, left iliac fossa pain, etc.

6) Diverticulitis has the same manifestations as ?

- Diverticulitis has the same manifestations as colon cancer.

7) What is the major difference between colon cancer and diverticulitis in their manifestations ?

- A major difference between colon cancer and diverticulitis in their manifestations is that diverticulitis is often accompanied by fever.

8) What is the surgical treatment for diverticulitis ?

- The surgical treatment for diverticulitis is the removal of the affected part of the colon.

9) What is the non-surgical and non-medicated treatment for diverticulitis ?

- A strict diet is a non-surgical and non-medicated treatment for diverticulitis.

10) What are some medication treatments for diverticulitis ?

- Some medication treatments for diverticulitis include treatment for pain and antibiotics.

Chapter 6

1) Can diverticulitis lead to colon cancer ?

- Yes, diverticulitis can lead to colon cancer.

2) Why is a liquid diet usually used as treatment for a patient with diverticulitis ?

- A liquid diet is usually used as treatment for a patient with diverticulitis because it helps the colon rest for a couple of days.

3) Give examples of drugs that can lead to diverticulitis.

- Corticosteroids can lead to diverticulitis.

4) Which kind of diverticulum is usually in an adult population ?

- False diverticulum is usually in an adult population.

5) Which kind of diverticulum is usually in the young children population ?

- True diverticulum is usually in the young children population.

6) Why is the false diverticulum usually in the adult population ?

- The false diverticulum is usually in the adult population because this type of diverticulum is acquired.

7) Why is true diverticulum usually in the young children population ?

- True diverticulum is usually in the young children population because it is hereditary.

Chapter 7

1) What is colostomy ?

- Colostomy is the opening of a part of the colon to the skin.

2) What is the purpose of colostomy ?

- Colostomy enables the elimination of feces.

3) What are the complications of colostomy ?

- The complications of colostomy are necrosis, stoma retraction, stenosis, bleeding, peristomal fistula, prolapse, incisional hernia, peristomal abscess, bowel obstruction and hemorrhage stoma.

4) What is a fistula ?

- A fistula is a tear.

5) What is stenosis ?

- Stenosis is the shrinkage of a surface (tissue, body).

6) What is necrosis ?

- Necrosis is the death of a cell or tissue.

7) What is a retraction ?

-   A retraction is when a surface becomes smaller
    by contraction.

8) What is prolapse ?

-   Prolapse is the abnormal descent of an organ or
    a part of an organ.

9) What is a bowel obstruction ?

-   A bowel obstruction is a partial or a complete
    blockage of the intestinal transit.

10) What is a stoma ?

-   A stoma is a temporary or permanent opening in
    the body.

Chapter 8

1) What is an acute abdomen ?

- An acute abdomen is a swollen and tense abdomen.

2) What is septicemia ?

- Septicemia is a serious bloodstream infection.

3) Give another name for septicemia.

- Septicemia is also called sepsis.

4) What is a serious complication of sepsis ?

- A serious complication of sepsis is death.

5) What substances could be found in large quantities in the stool ?

- Bacteria could be found in large quantities in the stool.

6) What is a normal transit ?

- A normal transit is the presence of gas, stool, and peristalsis.

7) What is peristalsis ?

- Peristalsis is the symmetrical contraction and relaxation of the muscles of the digestive tract.

8) Is peristalsis a voluntary or an involuntary action?

-    Peristalsis is an involuntary action.

9) What are the signs of peristalsis ?

-    The signs of peristalsis are gas and stool.

10) What is fistula in an organ ?

-    A fistula is an opening from one passage to
     another in an organ.

Chapter 9

1) What are the main functions of leukocytes ?

- Leukocytes protect the body against infections and foreign bodies.

2) Does an increase in leukocyte mean an infection?

- No, an increase in leukocyte does not necessarily mean an infection.

3) What does an increase in leukocyte signify ?

- An increase in leukocyte signifies inflammation.

4) What does an increase in protein C signify ?

- An increase in protein C signifies an infection.

5) What does it signify when leukocytes and CRP increase ?

- An increase in leukocytes and CRP signifies an infection.

6) How is the glucose level during fever ?

- There is a decrease in glucose level during fever because there is a decrease in metabolism since the body uses energy to fight the fever.

7) What can happen if a fever exceeds 40 degrees?

- A convulsion may occur if the temperature exceeds 40 degrees in case of fever.

8) What is a common name for hemorrhage ?

- A common name for hemorrhage is bleeding.

9) Define blood pressure.

- Blood pressure is the pressure that blood exerts on the walls of the arteries.

10) What is a pulse ?

- A pulse represents the regular beat of blood caused by the contraction of the heart.

Chapter 10

1) Is blood pressure high or low during hemorrhage?

- Blood pressure is low during hemorrhage.

2) Is the pulse high or low during hemorrhage ?

- The pulse is high during hemorrhage.

3) What are the steps in an abdominal evaluation ?

- The steps in an abdominal evaluation are inspection, palpation, auscultation, and percussion.

4) What does it mean when there is no sound during an abdominal auscultation ?

- The absence of sound during an abdominal auscultation is an alarm signal because there is no intestinal movement.

5) How long do contents stay in the large intestine ?

- Contents stay in the large intestine from 12 to 24 hours.

6) Is the defecation reflex sympathetic or parasympathetic ?

- The defecation reflex is sympathetic.

7) What is a skeletal muscle ?

- A skeletal muscle is a voluntary muscle. It is a muscle that we can control.

8) What is a smooth muscle ?

- A smooth muscle is an involuntary muscle. It is a muscle that we cannot control.

9) What kind of muscle is the internal sphincter of the anus ?

- The internal sphincter of the anus is a smooth muscle.

10) What kind of muscle is the external sphincter of the anus ?

- The external sphincter of the anus is a skeletal muscle.

11) Name a unique skeletal muscle that is involuntary in the body.

- The heart muscle is a unique muscle that is a skeletal muscle but involuntary.

12) Is the colon an indispensable organ ?

- No, the colon is not an indispensable organ. A person can live without the colon.

13) What is the structure that prevents contents from returning to the small intestine after they have entered the large intestine ?

-   The ileocecal valve prevents contents from flowing back to the small intestine after they have entered the large intestine.

Conclusion

Thank you again for purchasing this book. I hope it has helped you in your journey to understanding Diverticulitis and how it affects the people around you who suffer from it.

Thank you.